111

Kettlebell

Workouts

Book for Men and Women

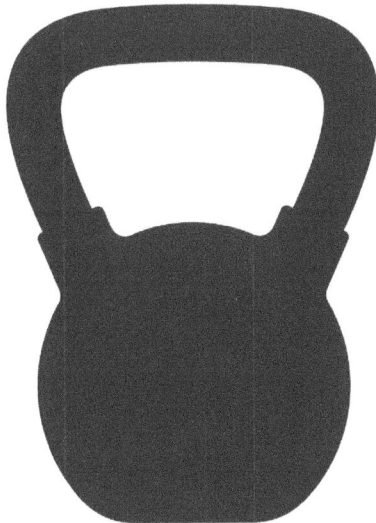

111
Kettlebell
Workouts
Book for Men and Women

111 Workouts to
Build Muscle and Lose Fat

Extra Logging Sheets & Videos to Watch
Exercises
Are Available by Scanning QR Codes

Be.Bull Publishing Group

Toronto, Canada

Authors:

Be.Bull Publishing Group

Devon Abbruzzese & Mauricio Vasquez

First Printing: July 2022

ISBN- 978-1-990709-50-0

FREE DOWNLOAD

BONUS No 1

ALL LOGGING SHEETS from this book are available *FOR NO EXTRA COST* for you by scanning a QR code.

You can scan the QR code, print, and record your workouts to measure your performance as many times as you want.

(The QR is found at the end of this book)

BONUS No 2 -

VIDEOS for ALL EXERCISES ARE AVAILABLE to check how the exercises are to be performed

(The QR codes are found at the end of this book)

Unlock Your Fitness Potential
with Artificial Intelligence

I am thrilled to introduce a groundbreaking tool, *"AI-Powered Training Coach" GPT*, for physical fitness, developed with the latest advancements in AI technology. This advanced tool is designed to enhance your workout experience, offering personalized exercise plans tailored to your preferences, needs, and the equipment you have available.

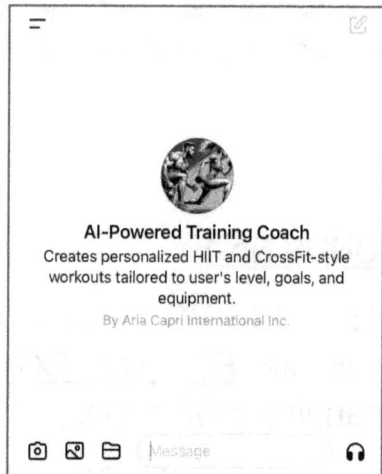

AI-Powered Training Coach
Creates personalized HIIT and CrossFit-style workouts tailored to user's level, goals, and equipment.
By Aria Capri International Inc.

This innovative AI system, utilizing Generative Pre-trained Transformer (GPT) technology by OpenAI.com, is specifically programmed to support your fitness journey. It acts as a dynamic fitness companion, aligning with your personal fitness goals and the resources at your disposal, providing custom-tailored workout routines and fitness advice.

Engaging with this AI tool is incredibly user-friendly and intuitive. Upon access, you'll be presented with a straightforward interface where you can input your fitness objectives, available equipment, and other relevant details. The AI processes this information rapidly, delivering tailored workout plans and suggestions almost instantly.

Whether your goal is to build muscle, increase endurance, or simply maintain a healthy lifestyle, this AI tool is your gateway to a more effective and personalized fitness experience.

Included in this section there are a couple of screenshots displaying the user interface you'll encounter when accessing this unique fitness AI tool. This visual guide offers a clear overview of the tool's functionality, assisting you in your first steps towards a smarter, AI-enhanced workout regimen.

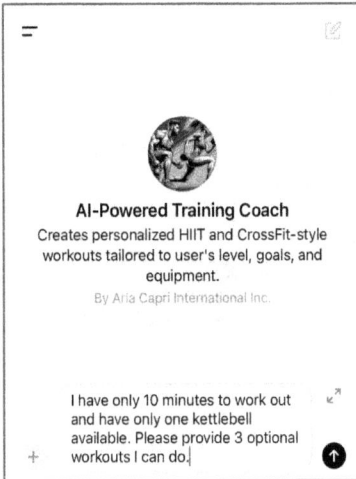

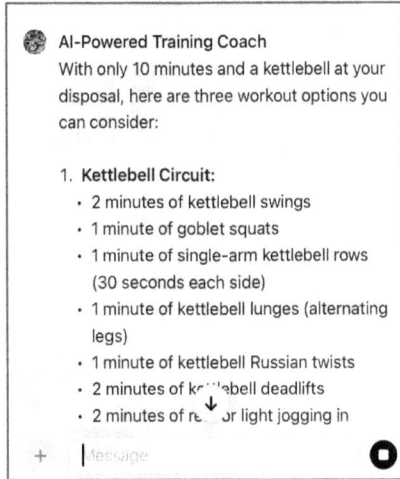

AI-Powered Training Coach
Creates personalized HIIT and CrossFit-style workouts tailored to user's level, goals, and equipment.
By Aria Capri International Inc.

I have only 10 minutes to work out and have only one kettlebell available. Please provide 3 optional workouts I can do.

AI-Powered Training Coach
With only 10 minutes and a kettlebell at your disposal, here are three workout options you can consider:

1. **Kettlebell Circuit:**
   - 2 minutes of kettlebell swings
   - 1 minute of goblet squats
   - 1 minute of single-arm kettlebell rows (30 seconds each side)
   - 1 minute of kettlebell lunges (alternating legs)
   - 1 minute of kettlebell Russian twists
   - 2 minutes of kettlebell deadlifts
   - 2 minutes of rest or light jogging in

To embark on your journey towards achieving your fitness goals with the support of this innovative AI technology, please go to this link
https://mindscapeartwork.ck.page/trainingcoachgpt
or scan this QR code.

Go to the link or scan the QR code shown below to check out other workout books

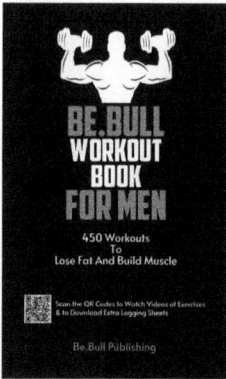

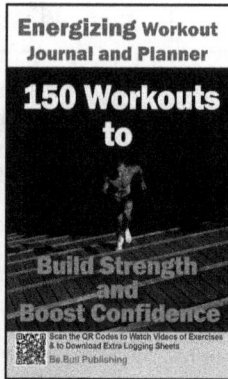

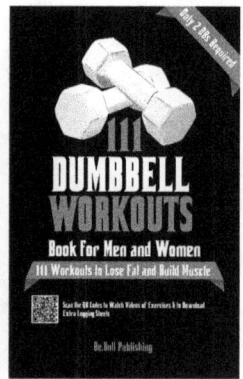

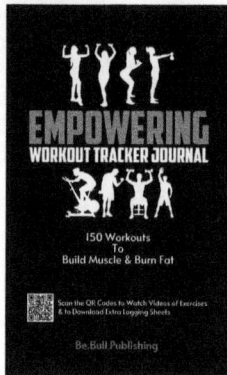

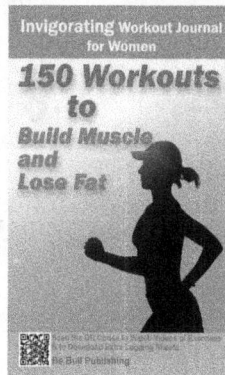

BE.BULL WORKOUT BOOK FOR MEN
450 Workouts To Lose Fat And Build Muscle
Scan the QR Codes to Watch Videos of Exercises & to Download Extra Logging Sheets
Be.Bull Publishing

Energizing Workout Journal and Planner
150 Workouts to Build Strength and Boost Confidence
Scan the QR Codes to Watch Videos of Exercises & to Download Extra Logging Sheets
Be.Bull Publishing

111 DUMBBELL WORKOUTS
Book For Men and Women
111 Workouts to Lose Fat and Build Muscle
Scan the QR Codes to Watch Videos of Exercises & to Download Extra Logging Sheets
Be.Bull Publishing

EMPOWERING WORKOUT TRACKER JOURNAL
150 Workouts To Build Muscle & Burn Fat
Scan the QR Codes to Watch Videos of Exercises & to Download Extra Logging Sheets
Be.Bull Publishing

Invigorating Workout Journal for Women
150 Workouts to Build Muscle and Lose Fat
Scan the QR Codes to Watch Videos of Exercises & to Download Extra Logging Sheets
Be.Bull Publishing

https://linktr.ee/be.bull

TIPS

- Adjust the weight of the kettlebell, the number of repetitions and the time cap for the workouts according to your capabilities, skills and physical condition
- Listen to your body and don't push yourself too hard
- If you don't have enough space where to run, you can do jumping jacks. 100-meter run is approximately equivalent to 50 jumping jacks
- Walk into the gym with a workout already selected for you
- Get motivated with a fun workout playlist
- Put your phone on airplane mode
- Start your workout with some stretches
- Pick the right weight - you will notice that the workouts don't indicate a specific weight. That is on purpose. Just choose a weight that is right for you.
- Log the details of each workout so you can track your progress. You can track the weight, time and number of repetitions
- Enjoy your workouts

Disclaimer

1. Be.Bull Publishing (Aria Capri International Inc.) strongly recommends that you consult with your physician before beginning any exercise program or workout. You should be in good physical condition and be able to participate in the exercises and workouts. We are not a licensed medical care provider and represents that we have no expertise in diagnosing, examining, or treating medical conditions of any kind, or in determining the effect of any specific exercise or workout on a medical condition.

2. You should understand that when participating in any exercise or workout, there is the possibility of physical injury. If you engage in the exercises and workouts of this book, you agree that you do so at your own risk, are voluntarily participating in these activities, assume all risk of injury to yourself, and agree to release and discharge Be.Bull Publishing (Aria Capri International Inc.) from any and all claims or causes of action, known or unknown, arising out of this book and videos.

3. The information provided through this book is not intended to be a substitute for professional medical advice, diagnosis or treatment. Never disregard professional medical advice, or delay in seeking it, because of something you have read on this book or watch in the videos. Never rely on information on this book or videos in place of seeking professional medical advice.

4. Be.Bull Publishing (Aria Capri International Inc.) is not responsible or liable for any advice, course of treatment, diagnosis or any other information, services or products that you obtain through this book or videos. You are encouraged to consult with your doctor with regard to the information contained on or through this book or videos. After reading this book or watching videos from this book, you are encouraged to review the information carefully with your professional healthcare provider.

WORKOUTS	Day 1 Reps / Time / Weight	Day 2 Reps / Time / Weight	Day 3 Reps / Time / Weight	Day 4 Reps / Time / Weight	Day 5 Reps / Time / Weight
1 2-minute Elbow Plank 10 Burpees 15 Kettlebell Swings 30 Push-Ups 45 Goblet Squats 45 Burpees 30 Kettlebell Swings 15 Push-Ups 10 Goblet Squats 2-minute Elbow Plank					
2 20 Turkish Get-Ups (Right Arm) 50 Kettlebell Swings 20 Overhead Squats (Left Arm) 50 Kettlebell Swings 20 Overhead Squats (Right Arm) 50 Kettlebell Swings 20 Turkish Get-Ups (Left Arm)					
3 5 Rounds for Time 25 Kettlebell Swings 500 meter Run					
4 50 Air Squats 15 Burpees 40 Sit-Ups 15 Burpees 30 Lunges (alternating legs) 15 Burpees 20 Kettlebell Swings 15 Burpees 10 meter Bear Crawl 15 Burpees 20 Kettlebell Swings 15 Burpees 30 Lunges (alternating legs) 15 Burpees 40 Sit-Ups 15 Burpees 50 Air Squats					

	Day 6	Day 7	Day 8	Day 9	Day 10
WORKOUTS	Reps / Time / Weight	Reps / Time / Weight	Reps / Time / Weight	Reps / Time / Weight	Reps / Time / Weight
1 2-minute Elbow Plank 10 Burpees 15 Kettlebell Swings 30 Push-Ups 45 Goblet Squats 45 Burpees 30 Kettlebell Swings 15 Push-Ups 10 Goblet Squats 2-minute Elbow Plank					
2 20 Turkish Get-Ups (Right Arm) 50 Kettlebell Swings 20 Overhead Squats (Left Arm) 50 Kettlebell Swings 20 Overhead Squats (Right Arm) 50 Kettlebell Swings 20 Turkish Get-Ups (Left Arm)					
3 5 Rounds for Time 25 Kettlebell Swings 500 meter Run					
4 50 Air Squats 15 Burpees 40 Sit-Ups 15 Burpees 30 Lunges (alternating legs) 15 Burpees 20 Kettlebell Swings 15 Burpees 10 meter Bear Crawl 15 Burpees 20 Kettlebell Swings 15 Burpees 30 Lunges (alternating legs) 15 Burpees 40 Sit-Ups 15 Burpees 50 Air Squats					

	WORKOUTS	Day 1 Reps / Time / Weight	Day 2 Reps / Time / Weight	Day 3 Reps / Time / Weight	Day 4 Reps / Time / Weight	Day 5 Reps / Time / Weight
5	21-15-9 Reps for Time Burpees Kettlebell Swings					
6	100 Air Squats 100 Kettlebell Swings 100 Sit-Ups 100 Push-Ups					
7	100 Kettlebell Swings 3 Burpees at the top of each minute					
8	25 Goblet Squats 50 Push-Ups 75 Sit-Ups 50 Russian Kettlebell Swings 25 Burpees					
9	10 Burpees 15 Push-Ups 25 Kettlebell Swings Buy-in: 70 Sit-Ups					
10	500 meter Run 50 Russian Kettlebell Swings 25 Air Squats					
11	10 Rounds for Time 10 Kettlebell Squats 10 Burpees 10 Kettlebell Swings 10 Pushups					
12	As many rounds as possible in 15 minutes: 25 Kettlebell Deadlifts 25 Air Squats 25 Situps					
13	Every minute on the minute for 10 minutes: Even minutes - 22 kettlebell swings Odd minutes - 11 burpees					

	WORKOUTS	Day 6 Reps / Time / Weight	Day 7 Reps / Time / Weight	Day 8 Reps / Time / Weight	Day 9 Reps / Time / Weight	Day 10 Reps / Time / Weight
5	21-15-9 Reps for Time Burpees Kettlebell Swings					
6	100 Air Squats 100 Kettlebell Swings 100 Sit-Ups 100 Push-Ups					
7	100 Kettlebell Swings 3 Burpees at the top of each minute					
8	25 Goblet Squats 50 Push-Ups 75 Sit-Ups 50 Russian Kettlebell Swings 25 Burpees					
9	10 Burpees 15 Push-Ups 25 Kettlebell Swings Buy-in: 70 Sit-Ups					
10	500 meter Run 50 Russian Kettlebell Swings 25 Air Squats					
11	10 Rounds for Time 10 Kettlebell Squats 10 Burpees 10 Kettlebell Swings 10 Pushups					
12	As many rounds as possible in 15 minutes: 25 Kettlebell Deadlifts 25 Air Squats 25 Situps					
13	Every minute on the minute for 10 minutes: Even minutes - 22 kettlebell swings Odd minutes - 11 burpees					

	WORKOUTS	Day 1 Reps / Time / Weight	Day 2 Reps / Time / Weight	Day 3 Reps / Time / Weight	Day 4 Reps / Time / Weight	Day 5 Reps / Time / Weight
14	500 meter Run 25 Push-Ups 50 Goblet Squats 500 meter Run 25 Push-Ups 50 Kettlebell Swings 500 meter Run					
15	As many rounds as possible in 25 minutes 5 Kettlebell Half Snatches (Right arm) 5 Kettlebell Half Snatches (Left arm) 5 Burpees 10 Kettlebell Deadlifts					
16	As many rounds as possible in 20 minutes: 10 Pushups 20 Kettlebell Squats 30 Mountain Climbers					
17	7 rounds per time of: 20 Air Squats 20 Kettlebell Deadlifts 20 V-ups 20 Push-ups					
18	4 Rounds for Time 24 Single-Arm Kettlebell Swings (split reps between arms) 24 Single-Arm Kettlebell Overhead Squats (split reps between arms) 24 Burpees 24 Push-ups					

		Day 6	Day 7	Day 8	Day 9	Day 10
	WORKOUTS	Reps / Time / Weight	Reps / Time / Weight	Reps / Time / Weight	Reps / Time / Weight	Reps / Time / Weight
14	500 meter Run 25 Push-Ups 50 Goblet Squats 500 meter Run 25 Push-Ups 50 Kettlebell Swings 500 meter Run					
15	As many rounds as possible in 25 minutes 5 Kettlebell Half Snatches (Right arm) 5 Kettlebell Half Snatches (Left arm) 5 Burpees 10 Kettlebell Deadlifts					
16	As many rounds as possible in 20 minutes: 10 Pushups 20 Kettlebell Squats 30 Mountain Climbers					
17	7 rounds per time of: 20 Air Squats 20 Kettlebell Deadlifts 20 V-ups 20 Push-ups					
18	4 Rounds for Time 24 Single-Arm Kettlebell Swings (split reps between arms) 24 Single-Arm Kettlebell Overhead Squats (split reps between arms) 24 Burpees 24 Push-ups					

	WORKOUTS	Day 1 Reps / Time / Weight	Day 2 Reps / Time / Weight	Day 3 Reps / Time / Weight	Day 4 Reps / Time / Weight	Day 5 Reps / Time / Weight
19	As many rounds as possible in 15 minutes Kettlebell Power Snatches					
20	21-19-17-15-13-11-9-7-5-3 Reps For Time of: Burpees American Kettlebell Swings					
21	15-13-11-9-7-5-3 Reps of: Kettlebell Snatches (each arm, alternating) After every round, perform: 5 Burpees 15 Prison Squats					
22	10 rounds of: 10 Kettlebell Squats 10 V-ups 10 Kettlebell Lunges					
23	500 meter Run 50 Russian Kettlebell Swings 50 Kettlebell Taters 400 meter Run 40 Russian Kettlebell Swings 40 Kettlebell Taters 300 meter Run 30 Russian Kettlebell Swings 30 Kettlebell Taters 200 meter Run 20 Russian Kettlebell Swings 20 Kettlebell Taters					

	WORKOUTS	Day 6 Reps / Time / Weight	Day 7 Reps / Time / Weight	Day 8 Reps / Time / Weight	Day 9 Reps / Time / Weight	Day 10 Reps / Time / Weight
19	As many rounds as possible in 15 minutes Kettlebell Power Snatches					
20	21-19-17-15-13-11-9-7-5-3 Reps For Time of: Burpees American Kettlebell Swings					
21	15-13-11-9-7-5-3 Reps of: Kettlebell Snatches (each arm, alternating) After every round, perform: 5 Burpees 15 Prison Squats					
22	10 rounds of: 10 Kettlebell Squats 10 V-ups 10 Kettlebell Lunges					
23	500 meter Run 50 Russian Kettlebell Swings 50 Kettlebell Taters 400 meter Run 40 Russian Kettlebell Swings 40 Kettlebell Taters 300 meter Run 30 Russian Kettlebell Swings 30 Kettlebell Taters 200 meter Run 20 Russian Kettlebell Swings 20 Kettlebell Taters					

WORKOUTS	Day 1 Reps / Time / Weight	Day 2 Reps / Time / Weight	Day 3 Reps / Time / Weight	Day 4 Reps / Time / Weight	Day 5 Reps / Time / Weight
24 500 meter Run 20 Kettlebell Swings 20 Burpees 20 Air Squats 20 Single-Arm Kettlebell Push Press (right arm) 500 meter Run 20 Kettlebell Swings 20 Burpees 20 Air Squats 20 Single-Arm Kettlebell Push Press (left arm) 500 meter Run					
25 As many rounds as possible in 18 minutes of: 3 Burpees 6 Kettlebell Swings 9 Kettlebell Squats					
26 As many rounds as possible in 25 minutes 15 Kettlebell Deadlifts 50 meter Kettlebell Farmer's Carry (Right arm) 15 Kettlebell Thrusters 50 meter Kettlebell Farmer's Carry (Left arm)					
27 As many rounds as possible in 15 minutes 3 Russian Kettlebell Swings 5 Burpees *Add 2 reps after each round					

		Day 6	Day 7	Day 8	Day 9	Day 10
WORKOUTS		Reps / Time / Weight	Reps / Time / Weight	Reps / Time / Weight	Reps / Time / Weight	Reps / Time / Weight
24	500 meter Run 20 Kettlebell Swings 20 Burpees 20 Air Squats 20 Single-Arm Kettlebell Push Press (right arm) 500 meter Run 20 Kettlebell Swings 20 Burpees 20 Air Squats 20 Single-Arm Kettlebell Push Press (left arm) 500 meter Run					
25	As many rounds as possible in 18 minutes of: 3 Burpees 6 Kettlebell Swings 9 Kettlebell Squats					
26	As many rounds as possible in 25 minutes 15 Kettlebell Deadlifts 50 meter Kettlebell Farmer's Carry (Right arm) 15 Kettlebell Thrusters 50 meter Kettlebell Farmer's Carry (Left arm)					
27	As many rounds as possible in 15 minutes 3 Russian Kettlebell Swings 5 Burpees *Add 2 reps after each round					

	Day 1	Day 2	Day 3	Day 4	Day 5
WORKOUTS	Reps / Time / Weight	Reps / Time / Weight	Reps / Time / Weight	Reps / Time / Weight	Reps / Time / Weight
28 5 Russian Kettlebell Swings 50 meter Kettlebell Farmer's Carry (Right arm) 50 meter Kettlebell Farmer's Carry (Left arm) 10 Alternating Single-Arm Kettlebell Swings 20 American Kettlebell Swings 50 meter Kettlebell Farmer's Carry (Right arm) 50 meter Kettlebell Farmer's Carry (Left arm) 10 Left-Arm Kettlebell Swings 10 Right-Arm Kettlebell Swings 50 Russian Kettlebell Swings					
29 50 Kettlebell Deadlifts 50 Pushups 50 Kettlebell Squats 50 Burpees 50 Kettlebell Swings					
30 6 Rounds For Time: 12 Kettlebell Rows (split reps between arms) 10 Push-Ups 12 Goblet Squats 12 Kettlebell Swings					

	Day 6	Day 7	Day 8	Day 9	Day 10
WORKOUTS	Reps / Time / Weight	Reps / Time / Weight	Reps / Time / Weight	Reps / Time / Weight	Reps / Time / Weight
28 5 Russian Kettlebell Swings 50 meter Kettlebell Farmer's Carry (Right arm) 50 meter Kettlebell Farmer's Carry (Left arm) 10 Alternating Single-Arm Kettlebell Swings 20 American Kettlebell Swings 50 meter Kettlebell Farmer's Carry (Right arm) 50 meter Kettlebell Farmer's Carry (Left arm) 10 Left-Arm Kettlebell Swings 10 Right-Arm Kettlebell Swings 50 Russian Kettlebell Swings					
29 50 Kettlebell Deadlifts 50 Pushups 50 Kettlebell Squats 50 Burpees 50 Kettlebell Swings					
30 6 Rounds For Time: 12 Kettlebell Rows (split reps between arms) 10 Push-Ups 12 Goblet Squats 12 Kettlebell Swings					

WORKOUTS	Day 1 Reps / Time / Weight	Day 2 Reps / Time / Weight	Day 3 Reps / Time / Weight	Day 4 Reps / Time / Weight	Day 5 Reps / Time / Weight
31 500 meter Run 50 Kettlebell Single-Arm Hang Snatches (split reps between arms) 500 meter Run 50 Kettlebell Single-Arm Hang Clean and Push Presses (split reps between arms)					
32 As many rounds as possible in 15 minutes: 9 Sumo Deadlift High Pull 15 Goblet Squats 21 Kettlebell Swings					
33 For time: 20 Turkish Get-Ups (Right Arm) 60 Kettlebell Swings 20 Overhead Squats (Left Arm) 60 Kettlebell Swings 20 Overhead Squats (Right Arm) 60 Kettlebell Swings 20 Turkish Get-Ups (Left Arm)					
34 400 Air Squats 200 American Kettlebell Swings					
35 250 Russian Kettlebell Swings Every minute on the minute, perform Burpee(s). Start with 1 Burpee after minute 1, then 2 Burpees after minute 2, then 3 Burpees, etc. (Stop adding Burpees once you get less than 30 seconds left for your Swings)					

	Day 6	Day 7	Day 8	Day 9	Day 10
WORKOUTS	**Reps / Time / Weight**	**Reps / Time / Weight**	**Reps / Time / Weight**	**Reps / Time / Weight**	**Reps / Time / Weight**
31 500 meter Run 50 Kettlebell Single-Arm Hang Snatches (split reps between arms) 500 meter Run 50 Kettlebell Single-Arm Hang Clean and Push Presses (split reps between arms)					
32 As many rounds as possible in 15 minutes: 9 Sumo Deadlift High Pull 15 Goblet Squats 21 Kettlebell Swings					
33 For time: 20 Turkish Get-Ups (Right Arm) 60 Kettlebell Swings 20 Overhead Squats (Left Arm) 60 Kettlebell Swings 20 Overhead Squats (Right Arm) 60 Kettlebell Swings 20 Turkish Get-Ups (Left Arm)					
34 400 Air Squats 200 American Kettlebell Swings					
35 250 Russian Kettlebell Swings Every minute on the minute, perform Burpee(s). Start with 1 Burpee after minute 1, then 2 Burpees after minute 2, then 3 Burpees, etc. (Stop adding Burpees once you get less than 30 seconds left for your Swings)					

	WORKOUTS	Day 1 Reps / Time / Weight	Day 2 Reps / Time / Weight	Day 3 Reps / Time / Weight	Day 4 Reps / Time / Weight	Day 5 Reps / Time / Weight
36	As many rounds as possible in 15 minutes 5 Burpees 10 Single-Arm Kettlebell Snatches (Each arm) 20 Lunges (Alternating legs)					
37	4 Rounds For Time: 400m Run 21 Kettlebell Swings 15 Burpees					
38	20-18-16-14-12-10-8-6-4-2 reps of: Kettlebell Thrusters (split reps between arms) Burpees					
39	50-40-30-20-10 reps of: Push-Ups Kettlebell Swings					
40	As many rounds as possible in 20 minutes 500 meter Run 20 American Kettlebell Swings 15 Push-Ups 10 Burpees					
41	20-18-16-14-12-10-8 reps of: Kettlebell Thrusters (split reps between arms) Kettlebell Deadlifts					

	Day 6	Day 7	Day 8	Day 9	Day 10
WORKOUTS	Reps / Time / Weight	Reps / Time / Weight	Reps / Time / Weight	Reps / Time / Weight	Reps / Time / Weight
36	As many rounds as possible in 15 minutes 5 Burpees 10 Single-Arm Kettlebell Snatches (Each arm) 20 Lunges (Alternating legs)				
37	4 Rounds For Time: 400m Run 21 Kettlebell Swings 15 Burpees				
38	20-18-16-14-12-10-8-6-4-2 reps of: Kettlebell Thrusters (split reps between arms) Burpees				
39	50-40-30-20-10 reps of: Push-Ups Kettlebell Swings				
40	As many rounds as possible in 20 minutes 500 meter Run 20 American Kettlebell Swings 15 Push-Ups 10 Burpees				
41	20-18-16-14-12-10-8 reps of: Kettlebell Thrusters (split reps between arms) Kettlebell Deadlifts				

	Day 1	Day 2	Day 3	Day 4	Day 5
WORKOUTS	**Reps / Time / Weight**	**Reps / Time / Weight**	**Reps / Time / Weight**	**Reps / Time / Weight**	**Reps / Time / Weight**
42 11-10-9-8-7-6-5-4-3-2-1-2-3-4-5-6-7-8-9-10 reps of: American Kettlebell Swings Burpees					
43 21-19-17-15-13-11-9-7-5-3 reps of: Kettlebell Taters 3-5-7-9-11-13-15-17-19-21 reps of: Burpees					
44 20 Rounds for Time 15 Kettlebell Swings 10 Burpees					
45 400 Kettlebell Swings 5 Burpees - every minute on the minute					
46 120 Kettlebell Swings 5 Burpees - every minute on the minute					
47 For Time: 50-40-30-20-10 Kettlebell Swings Kettlebell Goblet Squats					
48 As many rounds as possible in 15 minutes 6 Russian Kettlebell Swings 3 Burpees 6 Cossack Squats (alternating legs) 12 Russian Kettlebell Swings 6 Burpees 12 Cossack Squats Continue with this pattern, adding 6 Russian Kettlebell Swings, 3 Burpees, and 6 Cossack Squats each round.					

	WORKOUTS	Day 6 Reps / Time / Weight	Day 7 Reps / Time / Weight	Day 8 Reps / Time / Weight	Day 9 Reps / Time / Weight	Day 10 Reps / Time / Weight
42	11-10-9-8-7-6-5-4-3-2-1-2-3-4-5-6-7-8-9-10 reps of: American Kettlebell Swings Burpees					
43	21-19-17-15-13-11-9-7-5-3 reps of: Kettlebell Taters 3-5-7-9-11-13-15-17-19-21 reps of: Burpees					
44	20 Rounds for Time 15 Kettlebell Swings 10 Burpees					
45	400 Kettlebell Swings 5 Burpees - every minute on the minute					
46	120 Kettlebell Swings 5 Burpees - every minute on the minute					
47	For Time: 50-40-30-20-10 Kettlebell Swings Kettlebell Goblet Squats					
48	As many rounds as possible in 15 minutes 6 Russian Kettlebell Swings 3 Burpees 6 Cossack Squats (alternating legs) 12 Russian Kettlebell Swings 6 Burpees 12 Cossack Squats Continue with this pattern, adding 6 Russian Kettlebell Swings, 3 Burpees, and 6 Cossack Squats each round.					

WORKOUTS		Day 1 Reps / Time / Weight	Day 2 Reps / Time / Weight	Day 3 Reps / Time / Weight	Day 4 Reps / Time / Weight	Day 5 Reps / Time / Weight
49	10 Rounds for Time 15 Russian Kettlebell Swings 15 American Kettlebell Swings 10 Burpees					
50	10 Rounds for Time 15 Russian Kettlebell Swings 15 Push-Ups 5 Burpees					
51	As many rounds as possible in 25 minutes First, 50-40-30-20-10 reps For Time of: Push-Ups Kettlebell Swings Then, in the remaining time, as many rounds as possible of: Air Squats					
52	As many rounds as possible in 15 minutes: 20 Kettlebell Swings 15 Kettlebell Sumo Deadlift High Pulls 10 Kettlebell Goblet Squat Perform 5 hollow rocks every time you drop the kettlebell					
53	100-80-60-40-20 Kettlebell Swings 50-40-30-20-10 Air Squats 25-20-15-10-5 Burpees Alternating between kettlebell swings, air squats and burpees					

	Day 6	Day 7	Day 8	Day 9	Day 10
WORKOUTS	Reps / Time / Weight	Reps / Time / Weight	Reps / Time / Weight	Reps / Time / Weight	Reps / Time / Weight
49 10 Rounds for Time 15 Russian Kettlebell Swings 15 American Kettlebell Swings 10 Burpees					
50 10 Rounds for Time 15 Russian Kettlebell Swings 15 Push-Ups 5 Burpees					
51 As many rounds as possible in 25 minutes First, 50-40-30-20-10 reps For Time of: Push-Ups Kettlebell Swings Then, in the remaining time, as many rounds as possible of: Air Squats					
52 As many rounds as possible in 15 minutes: 20 Kettlebell Swings 15 Kettlebell Sumo Deadlift High Pulls 10 Kettlebell Goblet Squat Perform 5 hollow rocks every time you drop the kettlebell					
53 100-80-60-40-20 Kettlebell Swings 50-40-30-20-10 Air Squats 25-20-15-10-5 Burpees Alternating between kettlebell swings, air squats and burpees					

	WORKOUTS	Day 1 Reps / Time / Weight	Day 2 Reps / Time / Weight	Day 3 Reps / Time / Weight	Day 4 Reps / Time / Weight	Day 5 Reps / Time / Weight
54	Every minute on the minute - 12 MINUTES Odd minute: 10 Kettlebell Thrusters (split reps between arms) Even minute: 20 American Kettlebell Swings					
55	5 Rounds For Time: 22 Kettlebell Swings 16 Kettlebell Power Cleans 10 Burpees					
56	10 Kettlebell Snatches (Right-Arm) 10 Burpees 10 Kettlebell Snatches (Left-Arm) 30 Air Squats 15 Kettlebell Push Jerks (Right-Arm) 15 Burpees 15 Kettlebell Push Jerks (Left-Arm) 45 Air Squats 20 Kettlebell Cleans (Right-Arm) 20 Burpees 20 Kettlebell Cleans (Left-Arm) 60 Air Squats					
57	100 Air Squats 80 Kettlebell Swings 20 Push-Ups 20 Air Squats 60 Kettlebell Swings 20 Push-Ups 40 Air Squats 40 Kettlebell Swings 20 Push-Ups 60 Air Squats 20 Kettlebell Swings 20 Push-Ups 80 Air Squats					

	WORKOUTS	Day 6 Reps / Time / Weight	Day 7 Reps / Time / Weight	Day 8 Reps / Time / Weight	Day 9 Reps / Time / Weight	Day 10 Reps / Time / Weight
54	Every minute on the minute - 12 MINUTES Odd minute: 10 Kettlebell Thrusters (split reps between arms) Even minute: 20 American Kettlebell Swings					
55	5 Rounds For Time: 22 Kettlebell Swings 16 Kettlebell Power Cleans 10 Burpees					
56	10 Kettlebell Snatches (Right-Arm) 10 Burpees 10 Kettlebell Snatches (Left-Arm) 30 Air Squats 15 Kettlebell Push Jerks (Right-Arm) 15 Burpees 15 Kettlebell Push Jerks (Left-Arm) 45 Air Squats 20 Kettlebell Cleans (Right-Arm) 20 Burpees 20 Kettlebell Cleans (Left-Arm) 60 Air Squats					
57	100 Air Squats 80 Kettlebell Swings 20 Push-Ups 20 Air Squats 60 Kettlebell Swings 20 Push-Ups 40 Air Squats 40 Kettlebell Swings 20 Push-Ups 60 Air Squats 20 Kettlebell Swings 20 Push-Ups 80 Air Squats					

		Day 1	Day 2	Day 3	Day 4	Day 5
	WORKOUTS	**Reps / Time / Weight**	**Reps / Time / Weight**	**Reps / Time / Weight**	**Reps / Time / Weight**	**Reps / Time / Weight**
58	60 RussianKettlebell Swings 50 Air Squats 40 Hand-release push ups 50 American Kettlebell Swings 40 Lunges 30 Hand-release push ups 40 Russian Kettlebell Swings 30 Air Squats 20 Hand-release push ups 30 Kettlebell Swing Snatch (split reps between arms) 20 Plyo Lunges 10 Hand-release push ups					
59	For Time: 120 Air Squats 80 Kettlebell Swings 20 Push-Ups 60 Air Squats 20 Push-Ups 40 Kettlebell Swings 20 Push-Ups 30 Air Squats 20 Kettlebell Swings 20 Push-Ups 15 Air Squats 10 Kettlebell Swings 20 Push-Ups					
60	Buy-In: 25 Burpees Then 10 Rounds of: 20 Kettlebell Swings 20 Push-Ups 10 Goblet Squats					

	WORKOUTS	Day 6 Reps / Time / Weight	Day 7 Reps / Time / Weight	Day 8 Reps / Time / Weight	Day 9 Reps / Time / Weight	Day 10 Reps / Time / Weight
58	60 RussianKettlebell Swings 50 Air Squats 40 Hand-release push ups 50 American Kettlebell Swings 40 Lunges 30 Hand-release push ups 40 Russian Kettlebell Swings 30 Air Squats 20 Hand-release push ups 30 Kettlebell Swing Snatch (split reps between arms) 20 Plyo Lunges 10 Hand-release push ups					
59	For Time: 120 Air Squats 80 Kettlebell Swings 20 Push-Ups 60 Air Squats 20 Push-Ups 40 Kettlebell Swings 20 Push-Ups 30 Air Squats 20 Kettlebell Swings 20 Push-Ups 15 Air Squats 10 Kettlebell Swings 20 Push-Ups					
60	Buy-In: 25 Burpees Then 10 Rounds of: 20 Kettlebell Swings 20 Push-Ups 10 Goblet Squats					

	Day 1	Day 2	Day 3	Day 4	Day 5
WORKOUTS	Reps / Time / Weight	Reps / Time / Weight	Reps / Time / Weight	Reps / Time / Weight	Reps / Time / Weight
61 50 Russian Kettlebell Swings 20 Goblet Squats 50 Russian Kettlebell Swings 50 Kettlebell Ballistic Rows (split reps between arms) 20 Goblet Squats 50 Russian Kettlebell Swings 50 Kettlebell Push Presses (split reps between arms) 50 Russian Kettlebell Swings 20 Goblet Squats 50 Russian Kettlebell Swings					
62 18-15-12-9-6-3 reps of: Kettlebell Taters Kettlebell Over Burpees 50 meter Bear Crawl Shuttles					
63 For Time: 500 Kettlebell Goblet Squats Perform 10 Kettlebell Russian Twists every time you stop					
64 10-20-30-40-50-40-30-20-10 reps of: Air Squats Russian Kettlebell Swings					

	WORKOUTS	Day 6 Reps / Time / Weight	Day 7 Reps / Time / Weight	Day 8 Reps / Time / Weight	Day 9 Reps / Time / Weight	Day 10 Reps / Time / Weight
61	50 Russian Kettlebell Swings 20 Goblet Squats 50 Russian Kettlebell Swings 50 Kettlebell Ballistic Rows (split reps between arms) 20 Goblet Squats 50 Russian Kettlebell Swings 50 Kettlebell Push Presses (split reps between arms) 50 Russian Kettlebell Swings 20 Goblet Squats 50 Russian Kettlebell Swings					
62	18-15-12-9-6-3 reps of: Kettlebell Taters Kettlebell Over Burpees 50 meter Bear Crawl Shuttles					
63	For Time: 500 Kettlebell Goblet Squats Perform 10 Kettlebell Russian Twists every time you stop					
64	10-20-30-40-50-40-30-20-10 reps of: Air Squats Russian Kettlebell Swings					

	Day 1	Day 2	Day 3	Day 4	Day 5
WORKOUTS	Reps / Time / Weight	Reps / Time / Weight	Reps / Time / Weight	Reps / Time / Weight	Reps / Time / Weight
65 7 Rounds for Time 7 Double Kettlebell Deadlifts 7 Kettlebell Snatches (Right-Arm) 7 Kettlebell Snatches (Left-Arm) 7 meter Bear Crawl Kettlebell Drag (Forward move) 7 meter Bear Crawl Kettlebell Drag (Backward move)					
66 10-9-8-7-6-5-4-3-2-1 Kettlebell Overhead Squat (each arm) 2-4-6-8-10-12-14-16-18-20 Kettlebell Swings					
67 100 Goblet Squats Every break, perform: 10 Russian Twists with kettlebell					
68 5 Rounds for Time 15 Kettlebell Swings 15 Push-Ups 15 Burpees 100 meter run					

	WORKOUTS	Day 6 Reps / Time / Weight	Day 7 Reps / Time / Weight	Day 8 Reps / Time / Weight	Day 9 Reps / Time / Weight	Day 10 Reps / Time / Weight
65	7 Rounds for Time 7 Double Kettlebell Deadlifts 7 Kettlebell Snatches (Right-Arm) 7 Kettlebell Snatches (Left-Arm) 7 meter Bear Crawl Kettlebell Drag (Forward move) 7 meter Bear Crawl Kettlebell Drag (Backward move)					
66	10-9-8-7-6-5-4-3-2-1 Kettlebell Overhead Squat (each arm) 2-4-6-8-10-12-14-16-18-20 Kettlebell Swings					
67	100 Goblet Squats Every break, perform: 10 Russian Twists with kettlebell					
68	5 Rounds for Time 15 Kettlebell Swings 15 Push-Ups 15 Burpees 100 meter run					

	WORKOUTS	Day 1 Reps / Time / Weight	Day 2 Reps / Time / Weight	Day 3 Reps / Time / Weight	Day 4 Reps / Time / Weight	Day 5 Reps / Time / Weight
69	As many rounds as possible in 20 minutes 30 second Kettlebell Swings (Left-Arm) 30 second Kettlebell Swings (Right-Arm) 30 second Kettlebell Snatches (Left-Arm) 30 second Kettlebell Snatches (Right-Arm) 30 second Kettlebell Overhead Reverse Lunges (Left-Arm) 30 second Kettlebell Overhead Reverse Lunges (Right-Arm) 30 Push-Ups					
70	Every minute on the minute: Min 1: 10 Kettlebell Swings + 10 Hollow Rocks Min 2: 10 Kettlebell Goblet Squats + 10 Butterfly Sit Ups					
71	50-40-30-20-10 Russian Kettlebell Swings 25-20-15-10-5 Burpees					
72	5 Rounds for Time 20 Alternating Jumping Lunges 20 Russian Kettlebell Swings 20 Push-ups					
73	200 Kettlebell Russian Swing *Every Break 500-meter Run					

	WORKOUTS	Day 6 Reps / Time / Weight	Day 7 Reps / Time / Weight	Day 8 Reps / Time / Weight	Day 9 Reps / Time / Weight	Day 10 Reps / Time / Weight
69	As many rounds as possible in 20 minutes 30 second Kettlebell Swings (Left-Arm) 30 second Kettlebell Swings (Right-Arm) 30 second Kettlebell Snatches (Left-Arm) 30 second Kettlebell Snatches (Right-Arm) 30 second Kettlebell Overhead Reverse Lunges (Left-Arm) 30 second Kettlebell Overhead Reverse Lunges (Right-Arm) 30 Push-Ups					
70	Every minute on the minute: Min 1: 10 Kettlebell Swings + 10 Hollow Rocks Min 2: 10 Kettlebell Goblet Squats + 10 Butterfly Sit Ups					
71	50-40-30-20-10 Russian Kettlebell Swings 25-20-15-10-5 Burpees					
72	5 Rounds for Time 20 Alternating Jumping Lunges 20 Russian Kettlebell Swings 20 Push-ups					
73	200 Kettlebell Russian Swing *Every Break 500-meter Run					

	Day 1	Day 2	Day 3	Day 4	Day 5
WORKOUTS	Reps / Time / Weight	Reps / Time / Weight	Reps / Time / Weight	Reps / Time / Weight	Reps / Time / Weight
74 50-40-30-20-10 of Kettlebell Swings 50 meters Bear Crawl 50 meters Reverse Bear Crawl					
75 10 rounds 10 Kettlebell Russian Swings 10 Air squats 3 Kettlebell Thrusters (Each arm)					
76 6 Rounds For Time: 12 Kettlebell Deadlifts 9 Kettlebell Cleans (Each arm) 6 Kettlebell Push Jerk (Each arm)					
77 10-20-30-40-50 reps Kettlebell Snatch (split reps between arms) *After each round 10 Burpees over Kettlebell					
78 For Time 20 Turkish Get-Ups (Right Arm) 50 Kettlebell Swings 20 Overhead Squats (Left Arm) 50 Kettlebell Swings 20 Overhead Squats (Right Arm) 50 Kettlebell Swings 20 Turkish Get-Ups (Left Arm)					

	Day 6	Day 7	Day 8	Day 9	Day 10
WORKOUTS	Reps / Time / Weight	Reps / Time / Weight	Reps / Time / Weight	Reps / Time / Weight	Reps / Time / Weight
74 50-40-30-20-10 of Kettlebell Swings 50 meters Bear Crawl 50 meters Reverse Bear Crawl					
75 10 rounds 10 Kettlebell Russian Swings 10 Air squats 3 Kettlebell Thrusters (Each arm)					
76 6 Rounds For Time: 12 Kettlebell Deadlifts 9 Kettlebell Cleans (Each arm) 6 Kettlebell Push Jerk (Each arm)					
77 10-20-30-40-50 reps Kettlebell Snatch (split reps between arms) *After each round 10 Burpees over Kettlebell					
78 For Time 20 Turkish Get-Ups (Right Arm) 50 Kettlebell Swings 20 Overhead Squats (Left Arm) 50 Kettlebell Swings 20 Overhead Squats (Right Arm) 50 Kettlebell Swings 20 Turkish Get-Ups (Left Arm)					

		Day 1	Day 2	Day 3	Day 4	Day 5
	WORKOUTS	Reps / Time / Weight	Reps / Time / Weight	Reps / Time / Weight	Reps / Time / Weight	Reps / Time / Weight
79	For Time: 100 Kettlebell Swings 100 Air Squats 100 Push-Ups 100 Sit-Ups					
80	10 Kettlebell Turkish Get-Ups (split reps between arms) 40 Kettlebell Sumo Deadlift High-Pulls 40 Kettlebell Cleans (split reps between arms) 40 Kettlebell Jerks (split reps between arms) 100-meter Kettlebell Waiter Carry 40 Kettlebell Figure 8 through Legs 40 American Kettlebell Swings 40 Kettlebell Deadlifts					
81	100 Air Squats 50 Kettlebell Sit-Ups 50 American Kettlebell Swings (split reps between arms) 50 Kettlebell Goblet Squats 100 meter Kettlebell Lunges 50 Kettlebell Bent Over Rows (split reps between arms) 50 American Kettlebell Swings (split reps between arms) 50 Kettlebell Snatches (split reps between arms)					

	WORKOUTS	Day 6 Reps / Time / Weight	Day 7 Reps / Time / Weight	Day 8 Reps / Time / Weight	Day 9 Reps / Time / Weight	Day 10 Reps / Time / Weight
79	For Time: 100 Kettlebell Swings 100 Air Squats 100 Push-Ups 100 Sit-Ups					
80	10 Kettlebell Turkish Get-Ups (split reps between arms) 40 Kettlebell Sumo Deadlift High-Pulls 40 Kettlebell Cleans (split reps between arms) 40 Kettlebell Jerks (split reps between arms) 100-meter Kettlebell Waiter Carry 40 Kettlebell Figure 8 through Legs 40 American Kettlebell Swings 40 Kettlebell Deadlifts					
81	100 Air Squats 50 Kettlebell Sit-Ups 50 American Kettlebell Swings (split reps between arms) 50 Kettlebell Goblet Squats 100 meter Kettlebell Lunges 50 Kettlebell Bent Over Rows (split reps between arms) 50 American Kettlebell Swings (split reps between arms) 50 Kettlebell Snatches (split reps between arms)					

	Day 1	Day 2	Day 3	Day 4	Day 5
WORKOUTS	Reps / Time / Weight	Reps / Time / Weight	Reps / Time / Weight	Reps / Time / Weight	Reps / Time / Weight
82 10 Push-Ups 30 Kettlebell Swings 9 Push-Ups 30 Kettlebell Swings 8 Push-Ups 30 Kettlebell Swings 7 Push-Ups 30 Kettlebell Swings 6 Push-Up 30 Kettlebell Swings					
83 3 Rounds for Time 50 meter Farmer's Carry (split reps between arms) 25 meter Walking Lunges 25 Kettlebell Swings 25 Goblet Squats Time Cap: 25 minutes					
84 20 Rounds 6 Kettlebell Swing 6 Kettlebell Clean and Push Jerk (split reps between arms) 10 Burpees 10 Kettlebell Russian Swings					
85 5 Rounds for Time: 800 meter Run 60 Russian Kettlebell Swings 40 Air Squats					
86 20-18-16-14-12-10-8-6-4-2 Reps For Time of Burpees Kettlebell Thrusters (Slit reps between arms) Burpees Kettlebell Sumo Deadlift High-Pulls Burpees Kettlebell Swings					

	WORKOUTS	Day 6 Reps / Time / Weight	Day 7 Reps / Time / Weight	Day 8 Reps / Time / Weight	Day 9 Reps / Time / Weight	Day 10 Reps / Time / Weight
82	10 Push-Ups 30 Kettlebell Swings 9 Push-Ups 30 Kettlebell Swings 8 Push-Ups 30 Kettlebell Swings 7 Push-Ups 30 Kettlebell Swings 6 Push-Up 30 Kettlebell Swings					
83	3 Rounds for Time 50 meter Farmer's Carry (split reps between arms) 25 meter Walking Lunges 25 Kettlebell Swings 25 Goblet Squats Time Cap: 25 minutes					
84	20 Rounds 6 Kettlebell Swing 6 Kettlebell Clean and Push Jerk (split reps between arms) 10 Burpees 10 Kettlebell Russian Swings					
85	5 Rounds for Time: 800 meter Run 60 Russian Kettlebell Swings 40 Air Squats					
86	20-18-16-14-12-10-8-6-4-2 Reps For Time of Burpees Kettlebell Thrusters (Slit reps between arms) Burpees Kettlebell Sumo Deadlift High-Pulls Burpees Kettlebell Swings					

WORKOUTS	Day 1 Reps / Time / Weight	Day 2 Reps / Time / Weight	Day 3 Reps / Time / Weight	Day 4 Reps / Time / Weight	Day 5 Reps / Time / Weight
87 10 Rounds 8 Kettlebell Clean (Split reps between arms) 8 Burpees 10 Air Squats					
88 5 Rounds for Time 500 meter Run 50 Walking Lunges 40 Sit-Ups 25 Push-Ups 40 Kettlebell Swings 10 Burpees Over Kettlebell					
89 300 Kettlebell Swings *Every minute on the minute: 5 Burpees starting at 01:00					
90 20-16-12-8-4 reps Kettlebell Cleans (Alternating arms) Hand Release Push Ups Burpees					
91 For Time 200 Russian Kettlebell Swings 100 American Kettlebell Swings Perform the following every time you put the kettlebell down: 15 Air Squats 10 Push-Ups 5 Burpees					

		Day 6	Day 7	Day 8	Day 9	Day 10
	WORKOUTS	**Reps / Time / Weight**	**Reps / Time / Weight**	**Reps / Time / Weight**	**Reps / Time / Weight**	**Reps / Time / Weight**
87	10 Rounds 8 Kettlebell Clean (Split reps between arms) 8 Burpees 10 Air Squats					
88	5 Rounds for Time 500 meter Run 50 Walking Lunges 40 Sit-Ups 25 Push-Ups 40 Kettlebell Swings 10 Burpees Over Kettlebell					
89	300 Kettlebell Swings *Every minute on the minute: 5 Burpees starting at 01:00					
90	20-16-12-8-4 reps Kettlebell Cleans (Alternating arms) Hand Release Push Ups Burpees					
91	For Time 200 Russian Kettlebell Swings 100 American Kettlebell Swings Perform the following every time you put the kettlebell down: 15 Air Squats 10 Push-Ups 5 Burpees					

	WORKOUTS	Day 1 Reps / Time / Weight	Day 2 Reps / Time / Weight	Day 3 Reps / Time / Weight	Day 4 Reps / Time / Weight	Day 5 Reps / Time / Weight
92	800 meter Run 30 Kettlebell Snatches 30 Kettlebell Clean and Push Jerk 30 Air Squats 30 Kettlebell Swings 30 V-ups 30 Burpees 30 Air Squats 30 Push-Ups 30 V-ups 30 Kettlebell Swings					
93	As many rounds as possible in 15 minutes 2 Russian Kettlebell Swings 4 Burpees					
94	20 min As many rounds as possible 10 Kettlebell Deadlifts 10 Push-ups 100m-run 20 Kettlebell Russian Swings					
95	5 Rounds for Time 25 Kettlebell Swings 500 meter Run					
96	5 Rounds of: 20 Push-ups 16 Kettlebell Snatches (Split reps between arms) 16 Kettlebell Push Press (Split reps between arms) 16 Kettlebell Snatches (Split reps between arms) 16 Kettlebell Push Press (Split reps between arms) 20 Push-ups					

WORKOUTS		Day 6 Reps / Time / Weight	Day 7 Reps / Time / Weight	Day 8 Reps / Time / Weight	Day 9 Reps / Time / Weight	Day 10 Reps / Time / Weight
92	800 meter Run 30 Kettlebell Snatches 30 Kettlebell Clean and Push Jerk 30 Air Squats 30 Kettlebell Swings 30 V-ups 30 Burpees 30 Air Squats 30 Push-Ups 30 V-ups 30 Kettlebell Swings					
93	As many rounds as possible in 15 minutes 2 Russian Kettlebell Swings 4 Burpees					
94	20 min As many rounds as possible 10 Kettlebell Deadlifts 10 Push-ups 100m-run 20 Kettlebell Russian Swings					
95	5 Rounds for Time 25 Kettlebell Swings 500 meter Run					
96	5 Rounds of: 20 Push-ups 16 Kettlebell Snatches (Split reps between arms) 16 Kettlebell Push Press (Split reps between arms) 16 Kettlebell Snatches (Split reps between arms) 16 Kettlebell Push Press (Split reps between arms) 20 Push-ups					

		Day 1	Day 2	Day 3	Day 4	Day 5
	WORKOUTS	Reps / Time / Weight	Reps / Time / Weight	Reps / Time / Weight	Reps / Time / Weight	Reps / Time / Weight
97	24 Russian Kettlebell Swings 24 Single Arm Kettlebell Suitcase Squats (Split reps between arms) 24 Sit-Ups 24 Kettlebell Snatches 24 Goblet Squats 24 Push-ups 24 American Kettlebell Swings					
98	As many rounds as possible in 15 min 5 Down ups 8 Kettlebell Thruster (Alternating arms) 11 Kettlebell Deadlifts 50m Kettlebell Goblet Carry					
99	20 Rounds for Time 6 Burpees 12 Goblet Squats 18 Kettlebell Swings 12 Burpees 6 Goblet Lunges (Alternating legs) 20 Push-Ups					
100	20 Push-up 10 Kettlebell Swing 20 Push-up 15 Kettlebell Swing 20 Push-up 25 Kettlebell Swing 20 Push-up 50 Kettlebell Swing					

	Day 6	Day 7	Day 8	Day 9	Day 10
WORKOUTS	Reps / Time / Weight	Reps / Time / Weight	Reps / Time / Weight	Reps / Time / Weight	Reps / Time / Weight
97 24 Russian Kettlebell Swings 24 Single Arm Kettlebell Suitcase Squats (Split reps between arms) 24 Sit-Ups 24 Kettlebell Snatches 24 Goblet Squats 24 Push-ups 24 American Kettlebell Swings					
98 As many rounds as possible in 15 min 5 Down ups 8 Kettlebell Thruster (Alternating arms) 11 Kettlebell Deadlifts 50m Kettlebell Goblet Carry					
99 20 Rounds for Time 6 Burpees 12 Goblet Squats 18 Kettlebell Swings 12 Burpees 6 Goblet Lunges (Alternating legs) 20 Push-Ups					
100 20 Push-up 10 Kettlebell Swing 20 Push-up 15 Kettlebell Swing 20 Push-up 25 Kettlebell Swing 20 Push-up 50 Kettlebell Swing					

WORKOUTS		Day 1 Reps / Time / Weight	Day 2 Reps / Time / Weight	Day 3 Reps / Time / Weight	Day 4 Reps / Time / Weight	Day 5 Reps / Time / Weight
101	20 Kettlebell Cossack Squat (Split reps between legs)					
	10 Kettlebell Swing					
	20 Kettlebell Cossack Squat (Split reps between legs)					
	15 Kettlebell Swing					
	20 Kettlebell Cossack Squat (Split reps between legs)					
	25 Kettlebell Swing					
	20 Kettlebell Cossack Squat (Split reps between legs)					
	50 Kettlebell Swing					
102	3 Rounds of: 20 Air Squats 20 Push-ups 20 Kettlebell Squat (Split reps between arms) 20 Kettlebell Swings (Split reps between arms)					
103	3 Rounds of: 400-meter Run 30 American Kettlebell Swings 20 Kettlebell Single Arm Front Rack Lunge (Split reps between arms) 10 Burpees Over Kettlebell 20 Kettlebell Thruster (Split reps between arms) 30 V Ups 400-meter Run					

		Day 6	Day 7	Day 8	Day 9	Day 10
WORKOUTS		**Reps / Time / Weight**	**Reps / Time / Weight**	**Reps / Time / Weight**	**Reps / Time / Weight**	**Reps / Time / Weight**
101	20 Kettlebell Cossack Squat (Split reps between legs) 10 Kettlebell Swing 20 Kettlebell Cossack Squat (Split reps between legs) 15 Kettlebell Swing 20 Kettlebell Cossack Squat (Split reps between legs) 25 Kettlebell Swing 20 Kettlebell Cossack Squat (Split reps between legs) 50 Kettlebell Swing					
102	3 Rounds of: 20 Air Squats 20 Push-ups 20 Kettlebell Squat (Split reps between arms) 20 Kettlebell Swings (Split reps between arms)					
103	3 Rounds of: 400-meter Run 30 American Kettlebell Swings 20 Kettlebell Single Arm Front Rack Lunge (Split reps between arms) 10 Burpees Over Kettlebell 20 Kettlebell Thruster (Split reps between arms) 30 V Ups 400-meter Run					

	WORKOUTS	Day 1 Reps / Time / Weight	Day 2 Reps / Time / Weight	Day 3 Reps / Time / Weight	Day 4 Reps / Time / Weight	Day 5 Reps / Time / Weight
104	50 Air Squats 10 Burpees 40 Sit-ups 10 Burpees 30 Kettlebell Clean Squat Press (Split reps between arms) 10 Burpees 20 Kettlebell Swings 10 Burpees 10 meter Bear Crawl 10 Burpees 20 Kettlebell Swings 10 Burpees 30 Kettlebell Clean Squat Press (Split reps between arms) 10 Burpees 40 Sit-ups 10 Burpees 50 Air Squats					
105	For Time of 50-40-30-20-10: Kettlebell Goblet Squats Kettlebell Swings					
106	Every minute on the minute for 12 minutes of: 25 Single Arm Kettlebell Swings (Right arm) 25 Single Arm Kettlebell Swings (Left arm) 8 Burpees					

	Day 6	Day 7	Day 8	Day 9	Day 10
WORKOUTS	**Reps / Time / Weight**	**Reps / Time / Weight**	**Reps / Time / Weight**	**Reps / Time / Weight**	**Reps / Time / Weight**
104	50 Air Squats 10 Burpees 40 Sit-ups 10 Burpees 30 Kettlebell Clean Squat Press (Split reps between arms) 10 Burpees 20 Kettlebell Swings 10 Burpees 10 meter Bear Crawl 10 Burpees 20 Kettlebell Swings 10 Burpees 30 Kettlebell Clean Squat Press (Split reps between arms) 10 Burpees 40 Sit-ups 10 Burpees 50 Air Squats					
105	For Time of 50-40-30-20-10: Kettlebell Goblet Squats Kettlebell Swings					
106	Every minute on the minute for 12 minutes of: 25 Single Arm Kettlebell Swings (Right arm) 25 Single Arm Kettlebell Swings (Left arm) 8 Burpees					

	WORKOUTS	Day 1	Day 2	Day 3	Day 4	Day 5
		Reps / Time / Weight	Reps / Time / Weight	Reps / Time / Weight	Reps / Time / Weight	Reps / Time / Weight
107	As many rounds as possible in 12 minutes of: 5 Kettlebell Clean and Press (Per arm) 5 Kettlebell Clean and Squat (Per arm) 6 Single-Arm Kettlebell Swings (Per arm) 6 Kettlebell Snatches (Per arm)					
108	6 Rounds of: 20 Kettlebell Swings 20 Burpees					
109	As many rounds as possible in 12 minutes of: 5 Burpees 10 Kettlebell Deadlifts 15 Goblet Squats 20 Kettlebell Swings					
110	For Time: 24 Kettlebell Clean Reverse Lunge (Alternating arms) 22 Kettlebell Push Press (Alternating arms) 20 Kettlebell Goblet Squat 18 Kettlebell V-Ups 16 Kettlebell Deadlift High-pulls					
111	As many rounds as possible in 22 minutos: 7 Burpees 14 Push-ups 28 Kettlebell Swings					

	WORKOUTS	Day 6 Reps / Time / Weight	Day 7 Reps / Time / Weight	Day 8 Reps / Time / Weight	Day 9 Reps / Time / Weight	Day 10 Reps / Time / Weight
107	As many rounds as possible in 12 minutes of: 5 Kettlebell Clean and Press (Per arm) 5 Kettlebell Clean and Squat (Per arm) 6 Single-Arm Kettlebell Swings (Per arm) 6 Kettlebell Snatches (Per arm)					
108	6 Rounds of: 20 Kettlebell Swings 20 Burpees					
109	As many rounds as possible in 12 minutes of: 5 Burpees 10 Kettlebell Deadlifts 15 Goblet Squats 20 Kettlebell Swings					
110	For Time: 24 Kettlebell Clean Reverse Lunge (Alternating arms) 22 Kettlebell Push Press (Alternating arms) 20 Kettlebell Goblet Squat 18 Kettlebell V-Ups 16 Kettlebell Deadlift High-pulls					
111	As many rounds as possible in 22 minutos: 7 Burpees 14 Push-ups 28 Kettlebell Swings					

BONUS No 1 - ALL LOGGING SHEETS of this book are available through this QR code that you can use to scan, print, and record your workouts to measure your performance as many times you want

Dear valued customer,

We are a small family-owned business, and we'd like to please kindly ask you to leave us a review.

We don't have the same budget as big publishing companies, so your support would be really appreciated. Your feedback will mean a lot to us, and we thank you in advance!

Mauricio & Devon

BONUS No 2 - VIDEOS for ALL EXERCISES ARE AVAILABLE HERE. If you want check how the exercises are to be performed, scan the QR codes with your mobile device.

Air Squats

Alternating Jumping Lunges

American Kettlebell Swings

Bear Crawl Kettlebell Drag

Bear Crawl Shuttles

Bear Crawl

Burpees

Down ups

Elbow Plank

Goblet Squats

Hand-release push ups

Hollow rocks

Kettlebell Clean and Press

Kettlebell Clean and Push Jerk

Kettlebell Clean and Squat

Kettlebell Clean and Strict Press

Kettlebell Clean
Reverse Lunge

Kettlebell Clean
Squat Press

Kettlebell Clean

Kettlebell
Clean-and-Jerk

Kettlebell Cossack
Squat

Kettlebell Deadlift

Kettlebell Farmer's
Carry

Kettlebell Goblet
Carry

Kettlebell Goblet
Squats

Kettlebell Half
Snatches

Kettlebell Lunges

Kettlebell Overhead
Reverse Lunges

Kettlebell Power
Cleans

Kettlebell Power
Snatches

Kettlebell Push
Jerks

Kettlebell Push
Press

Kettlebell Rows

Kettlebell Russian Twists

Kettlebell Single Arm Front Rack Lunge

Kettlebell Single-Arm Hang Clean and Push Presses

Kettlebell Single-Arm Hang Clean

Kettlebell Single-Arm Hang Snatches

Kettlebell Sit-Ups

Kettlebell Snatches

Kettlebell Squats

Kettlebell Strict Presses

Kettlebell Sumo Deadlift High-Pulls

Kettlebell Swing Snatch

Kettlebell Swings

Kettlebell Taters

Kettlebell Thruster

Kettlebell Turkish Get-Ups

Kettlebell V-Ups

Kettlebell
Waiter Carry

Lunges

Mountain Climbers

Overhead Squats

Plyo Lunges

Prison Squats

Push-Ups

Reverse Bear Crawl

Russian Kettlebell Swings

Russian Twists

Single Arm Kettlebell Suitcase Squats

Single-Arm Kettlebell Overhead Squats

Single-Arm Kettlebell Push Press

Single-Arm Kettlebell Swings

Sit-Ups

Turkish Get-Ups

V-ups